Holistic Healing

Discover Alternative Therapies and Wellness

Table of Contents

Chapter 1. Introduction

Embrace an exciting journey towards self-renewal and balance with this compelling Special Report, "Holistic Healing: Discover Alternative Therapies and Wellness." Immerse yourself in the welcoming world of holistic, natural approaches to health; learn about therapies that have been cherished by generations and innovative, novel techniques alike. This report engages you in a journey across the world and through the ages, bringing you in sync with the healing wisdom of nature. Whether you're a seasoned holistic practitioner or a curious newcomer, this report offers valuable insights for everyone – revealing secrets to the utmost well-being, happiness, and inner harmony. Get prepared to uplift your healing journey and explore the myriad paths to wellness that await you within this vibrant, inspiring Special Report. Step into wellness, let's make this beneficial discovery together!

Chapter 2. Exploring the Primal World of Holistic Healing

Holistic Healing is an exciting journey, filled with age-old wisdom from ancient cultures, combined with ever-advancing scientific discoveries. It spans a wide range of therapeutic methodologies, engaging every aspect of human life: physical, mental, emotional, and spiritual. Understanding its history and its potential for human health and wellbeing is an enlightening experience, one that stretches our awareness and broadens our perspectives about what health truly means. Let's embark on the exploration of this vast, primal world of holistic healing.

2.1. The Beginning of a Healing Journey

In every culture, throughout the ages, humans have sought ways to heal themselves and stay healthy. The earliest evidence of healing methods dates back to prehistory – the Stone Age – when early humans used plants and herbs as medicine. Many of these primal practices have been integrated into the healing methods we know as holistic healing today. These early humans intuitively knew that natural remedies could offer them health, restoration, and balance.

Archaeological evidence from various parts of the world supports the idea that ancient humans had a profound understanding of the healing properties of the natural world. They were skilled herbalists, with a profound knowledge of plants and their medicinal characteristics. The holistic approach of these ancient cultures influenced the development of holistic healing methods used today.

2.2. Holistic Healing in Ancient Cultures

Subsequent ages saw the development of a more organized system of healing in various parts of the world. The ancient Egyptians, for example, had a remarkable system of medicine which incorporated spirituality with healthcare. Ancient Egyptians believed that the divine could intervene in the healing process, showcasing one of the earliest examples of mind-body healing. Physical diseases were seen not just as physical problems, but also as spiritual disturbances.

Similarly, ancient Chinese medicine developed a holistic system aimed towards the balance of physical, emotional, and spiritual energies. Principles such as Yin and Yang, along with elements like Fire, Water, Wood, Metal, and Earth, became vital in understanding the human body, disease, and healing.

India's ancient healthcare system, Ayurveda, which is still in wide use today, believes in the balance of the body's Doshas - Vata, Pitta, and Kapha. Each individual is unique with a distinct combination of these three elements. Ayurveda offers personalized care, where treatments are based on a person's unique constitution, integrating diet, yoga, meditation, and herbal remedies as part of the healing process.

2.3. Emergence of Contemporary Holistic Healing

With the development of Western medicine in the modern age, the holistic practices of ancient cultures were overshadowed, but they never faded away completely. The late 20th century saw a resurgence of interest in holistic methodologies, emphasizing the importance of treating the whole person – body, mind, and spirit – rather than simply addressing the symptoms of illness.

Multiple therapies have re-emerged or been developed, encompassing a vast range of healing methods from nutrition, emotional freedom techniques, chiropractic care, homeopathy, to energy healing techniques such as Reiki and acupuncture, among others. These therapies may assist with various ailments, from physical pains to emotional traumas, thereby providing a more well-rounded health management approach.

2.4. The Unifying Principles of Holistic Healing

Regardless of the type of holistic therapy used, they all share a few common characteristics. These include:

- Recognition of the whole person – treating the whole individual, not just the symptoms of disease.

- The interconnectedness between mind, body, and spirit – understanding that these components are integral parts of the healing process.

- The power of self-healing – believing in the innate power of the body to heal itself, given the right conditions.

- The role of the practitioner as a guide – promoting the ideas of self-care, self-awareness, and individual responsibility for one's health.

These principles are what set holistic healing apart from conventional medical practices. They emphasize the need for individuals to take charge of their own health and to maintain balance in their lives.

2.5. The Future of Holistic Healing

With more and more people acknowledging the benefits of holistic healing, the future looks promising. Advances in scientific research are providing us insights into how these techniques work and revealing their effectiveness. Furthermore, combining these natural healing methods with advancements in Western medicine can potentially lead to more effective, personalized healthcare.

While we continue to explore and understand the primal world of holistic healing, we must remember the ancient wisdom that sparked its creation. The journey towards healing is deeply personal and individual, yet profoundly interconnected with our natural world. Only by understanding and respecting this association can we truly attain holistic health and wellness.

In the vast expanse of the Holistic Healing cosmos, new discoveries await. As we explore and learn more about this primitive yet innovative world, we are sure to unlock richer layers of our wellbeing. Uncover the secrets of the primal world of holistic healing, find what resonates with you, and begin your journey to balance and complete health.

Chapter 3. Connection of Mind, Body, and Spirit: The Triad of Holistic Approach

The complex relationship between mind, body, and spirit is recognized as vital in holistic practice. Nurturing all these three aspects can lead to an enhanced well-being. This chapter explores how these elements interweave to form the basis of holistic health, and discusses practices that promote harmony among them.

3.1. Understanding the Mind-Body-Spirit Connection

The analogy of mind, body, and spirit can be visualized like the three sides of a triangle. They interact and influence each other, crafting a balanced or imbalanced state of being. Meditative practices, physical exercises, and nurturing the spirit are ways holistic healing addresses this triad.

To understand this connection, it's vital to first address each part independently. The mind, often equated with intellect and consciousness, is the repository of our thoughts, beliefs, and emotions. Wounds of the mind can be as palpable as those of the body, evident in conditions such as depression or anxiety.

The body, our tangible shell, reveals signs of physical health or distress. The signs could be physiological, like pain or fatigue, or they can be external, as clear skin or weight changes.

The spirit, although more abstract, guides our motivations and values, our sense of purpose and connections with others. A troubled spirit could manifest in mood swings or feelings of emptiness.

3.2. Enriching the Mind: Positive Psychological Practices

Maintaining mental health is primarily about cultivating activities enhancing well-being. Mindfulness and meditation are such tools. They help gain self-awareness, lower stress and aid in acceptance of present surroundings.

Another practice is cognitive restructuring, which involves understanding our negative thought patterns and actively reshaping them into positives. Journaling is also beneficial – jotting down thoughts and feelings can provide release and insight.

3.3. Nurtifying the Body: Physical Wellness and Nutrition

Physical care works in tandem with mental practices. Physical movement aids in more efficient bodily functions, improved mood, and lower anxiety levels. It's important to engage in regular exercise that fits your lifestyle and interests. This could be yoga, swimming, cycling, or simply walking. Nutritious eating, adequate sleep, and regular health check-ups are also crucial.

Food is a key player in our bodily health. Eating a balanced, varied diet ensures the adequate intake of essential nutrients. Dietary practices can be diverse, from Mediterranean to vegan, but all should focus on the consumption of unprocessed foods.

3.4. Fostering the Spirit: Spiritual Nourishment

Spiritual health in a holistic sense isn't necessarily about religion. Rather, it's about our ability to connect – with ourselves, others, and the universe. Practices such as prayer, meditation, yoga, or spending time in nature can help nourish the spirit.

Engaging in activities that bring joy, comfort, or a sense of purpose can also bolster our spiritual health. Human connection is a crucial factor, so seek meaningful relationships and embrace community involvement.

3.5. The Intersection: How Mind, Body, and Spirit Cooperate

Everyone can understand the impact of a troubled mind on a hale body, but the inverse is equally apparent. Prolonged physical ailments can breed negative thoughts or anxiety. Similarly, a distressed spirit can give rise to both mental and physical discomfort.

When mind, body, and spirit are in harmony, it manifests as peace, contentment, and a positive outlook on life. This is the essential goal of any holistic healing approach.

Traditionally, Eastern practices like yoga and Tai Chi aim at this equilibrium. Modern psychotherapy acknowledges that the mind-body interface significantly impacts overall health and well-being.

3.6. Building up a Balanced Triad: A Lifetime Endeavor

Working towards holistic wellness is a lifelong journey. It is about creating a balance and maintaining it, even when life's inevitable disruptions occur. The idea is to be patient and persistent with the process.

Though the path may look different for everyone, the destination of mental, physical, and spiritual harmony is shared. This connection between mind, body, and spirit forms an integral aspect of holistic health, serving as a bridge between ancient wisdom and modern wellness practices.

Unraveling this intricate network paints a more encompassing picture of health and healing. It amplifies the idea that we're not just an assembly of disparate parts, but a complex, interconnected whole. To nurture all these elements can lead to an enriched sense of self, resilient health, and deep contentment. Rather than shunning conventional medicine, it encourages an amalgamation of every healing technique at our disposal. Holistic health is not just about living longer, but living better.

Chapter 4. Nutritional Wellness: The Power of Wholesome Diets

A balanced diet, nature's treasure trove of nutritional wellness, is the cornerstone of holistic health. Scientific evidence increasingly supports the view that alterations in diet have strong effects, both positive and negative, on health throughout life. This chapter delves into the significance of wholesome diets for a complement to a holistic approach to health and wellness.

4.1. Nutrients and Their Role in Health

What we consume fuels our bodies, but not all fuels are created equal. Nutritional wellness revolves around understanding this vital connection and making mindful choices about the foods we eat.

4.1.1. Macronutrients

Macronutrients, namely carbohydrates, proteins, and fats, are essential for providing energy to the body.

Carbohydrates, primarily stored in the liver and muscles, serve as a particularly important energy source in our bodies. Whole grain cereals, vegetables, and fruits are excellent sources of healthy carbohydrates.

Proteins, formed by amino acids, carry out functions related to the growth, repair, and maintenance of tissues. Lean meats, dairy, eggs, pulses, and soy are good sources of this macronutrient.

Fats play vital roles in hormone production, nutrient absorption, and cellular health. Notably, unsaturated fats found in avocados, nuts, seeds, and oils can substantially benefit health when consumed in moderation.

4.1.2. Micronutrients

Vitamins and minerals, referred to as micronutrients, are vital for disease prevention and the sustained function of our bodies. They are required in smaller amounts compared to macronutrients, but their absence in our diet can lead to severe ailments. Various fruits, vegetables, whole grains, dairy, and proteins provide ample amounts of these essential micronutrients.

4.1.3. Water

Water is a crucial nutrient that makes up about 60% of the human body. It's responsible for crucial bodily functions like maintaining body temperature, removing wastes, and lubricating your joints. Staying hydrated should always be a dietary priority.

4.2. Wholesome Diets and Their Impact

The benefits of whole foods over highly processed ones are numerous. They contain more nutrients, fiber, and protective substances. The philosophy of nutritional wellness lies in embracing this approach.

4.2.1. Prevention of Diseases

Eating a wholesome diet rich in fruits, veggies, lean proteins, and healthy fats helps decrease the risk of chronic diseases like obesity, heart disease, diabetes, and cancer.

4.2.2. Optimal Brain Health

Scientific research links healthy diets rich in omega-3 fatty acids, B-vitamins, and antioxidants to better brain health, potentially slowing cognitive decline and promoting mental sharpness.

4.2.3. Enhanced Mood and Energy Levels

The vitamins and minerals found in whole foods like fruits, vegetables, and whole grains stimulate the production of chemicals in our brain known as neurotransmitters. These neurotransmitter levels can significantly impact mood and energy levels.

4.3. Achieving Nutritional Wellness

Nutritional wellness is not one-size-fits-all. It's about finding the balance that works best for you. Here are some strategies to guide you on this journey.

4.3.1. Balancing Your Plate

A balanced meal includes multiple food groups. Incorporate lean proteins, whole grains, fruits, vegetables, and healthy fats to ensure a mix of essential nutrients.

4.3.2. Portion Control

Understanding portion sizes is essential to maintaining a balanced diet. Overeating any food, even healthy ones, can lead to excessive calorie intake.

4.3.3. Mindful Eating

Paying attention to your eating habits and understanding hunger cues can promote healthier eating patterns. It's about appreciating the food and enjoying the experience of eating, all while providing nourishment to your body.

4.4. The Role of Supplementation

While a balanced diet should cover almost all of your nutritional needs, some people may require supplements – such as pregnant women, older adults, and people with certain health conditions. Remember, they should not replace a balanced diet but rather should serve as a complement when necessary.

4.5. Embracing Dietary Diversity

Different foods provide different types and amounts of key nutrients. Accordingly, consuming a variety of foods across and within each food group will ensure intake of sufficient amounts of all necessary nutrients.

In summary, the power of a wholesome diet extends beyond mere weight management. Rich in vital nutrients, they are instrumental in maintaining peak physical and mental health, aiding disease prevention, and ensuring overall wellness. By acknowledging and understanding the significance of nutritional wellness in our lives, we can begin to make more mindful decisions about what we consume, bringing us one step closer to achieving holistic health.

Chapter 5. Discovering Ancient Eastern Healing Practices

Eastern healing therapies encompass a broad range of practices that have roots in traditional Asian medical philosophies. These therapies continue to significantly influence modern medical approaches, with increasing interest noted in the Western world. Undeniably, these ancient practices have offered profound insight and innovative treatment modalities, often focusing on balance, energy, and the inseparable connection between physical and mental health.

5.1. Yin and Yang

An essential cornerstone of Eastern healing practices is the concept of Yin and Yang, a fundamental symbol of harmony and balance originating from ancient Chinese philosophy. In a perfect balance between Yin and Yang, the universe is said to be in harmony. These two forces, although seemingly opposing, are inherently interconnected and mutually supportive, just as day complements night or cold counters heat. This understanding is paramount in the various healing methods and underlying theories of Eastern medicine.

5.2. Acupuncture

One of the most recognized Chinese medicinal practices in the west, acupuncture, harks back more than 2000 years. It operates on the belief that the body's vital energy, called 'qi' (pronounced "chee"), flows along channels, the meridians, which reach every corner of the body. Disease or ailment is considered an imbalance or blockage of 'qi'. The acupuncturist's objective is to restore balance using fine needles that stimulate specific points along these meridians.

The World Health Organization has recognized acupuncture as an effective treatment for a variety of conditions, including chronic pain, gastrointestinal disorders, and stress-related conditions. Reputed for its anti-inflammatory and analgesic properties, acupuncture joins the growing arsenal of complements to standard Western medicine's symptom management regimes.

5.3. Chinese Herbal Medicine

Chinese herbal medicine operates under the principles of Yin and Yang and dates back to the Shennong era over 2000 years ago. Herbalists draw from an extensive materia medica comprising over 13,000 substances in the form of plants, minerals, and animal products to rebalance the body's energies, strengthening the body's natural defenses.

Many modern medicines, such as artemisinin for malaria and ephedrine for asthma, have roots in Chinese herbal medicine, proving its immense contribution to global health.

5.4. Indian Ayurveda

In the Indian subcontinent, the ancient system of medicine, known as Ayurveda, has been practiced for over 3000 years. As the name suggests (Ayur = life, Veda = knowledge), Ayurveda is significantly more than a mere healing system. It is a comprehensive way of life.

Ayurveda categorizes individuals into three doshas: Vata, Pitta, and Kapha, representing the elements air, fire, and earth-water, respectively. The balance of these doshas establishes a person's constitution, or 'Prakriti.' Imbalances may lead to illness. Therefore, treatment targets re-establishing the dosha balance using lifestyle changes, herbal therapies, and physical treatments such as massage.

Ayurveda has been influential in the Western world, especially in the realm of diet and lifestyle interventions, promoting mindful eating practices and powerful nutritional strategies to support overall health.

5.5. Yoga and Meditation

Originating from ancient India, yoga is a physical, mental, and spiritual discipline aiming to connect the body, mind, and spirit. Hatha, Ashtanga, Vinyasa, Kundalini, or Iyengar yoga are a few common types differing in postures, sequences, and intensity. Various studies have affirmed yoga's positive effects on mental health, flexibility, strength, and balance.

Likewise, meditation is an adjunct therapy often coupled with yoga, providing a suite of cognitive and emotional benefits. It is acknowledged for its power to reduce stress, anxiety, and depression, improving sleep quality and enhancing overall well-being.

5.6. Korean Medicine

Traditional Korean medicine shares similarities with Chinese medicine but boasts distinct techniques like Sasang typology. Sasang divides people into four constitutions, each requiring unique dietary and lifestyle adjustments to balance health. Herb-infused treatments, manual therapies and energy treatments form an integral part of this healing system as well.

5.7. Japanese Kampo Medicine

Kampo medicine, a Japanese adaptation of Chinese medicine, has received coverage under the national health system in Japan. Kampo uses a smaller selection of herbs, usually in pre-formulated combinations. The therapeutic applications range from chronic ailments such as allergy, asthma, and gastrointestinal issues to supporting the overall wellness of the body.

Eastern medicine emphasizes the prevention of disease by nurturing the body's resilience and strength. The integration of mind, body, and spirit remains central to these traditional therapies. By harnessing the ancient wisdom of Eastern practices, we could unlock untapped potentials for global health, permitting us to balance our modern lifestyle while nourishing health from all dimensions.

Chapter 6. Homeopathy and Flower Essences: Nature's Gentle Healers

Homeopathy, a medical philosophy and practice that originated in the late 18th century, conceptualizes health as a delicate balance of mind, body, and spirit. It respects each individual's unique response to illness and recognizes the root causes of disease as deeply interwoven with our mental, emotional, and physical states. Similarly, Flower Essences, developed in the 1930s by Dr. Edward Bach, are liquid infusions made from blossoms. They function on an energetic level, akin to homeopathy, to address imbalances in the emotional body, thus affecting physical health indirectly.

6.1. Homeopathy: A Brief History

Homeopathy was developed by Samuel Hahnemann, a German physician frustrated with the harmful medical practices of his era, which included bloodletting and purging. Hahnemann proposed a revolutionary theory - "like cures like." This was the principle similia similibus curentur, or "let likes be cured by likes." If a substance could induce symptoms in a healthy person, Hahnemann inferred, it could treat similar symptoms in a sick person.

Hahnemann began preparing medicines following a method now called "potentization," which involves sequential dilution and vigorous shaking, or succussion. When a substance is highly potentized, it moves into an energetic form that can stimulate our vital force to react.

6.2. Homeopathic Medicines: The Science and Philosophy

Homeopathic medicines are derived from various plant, mineral, and animal sources, undergoing a unique method of preparation. Substances are diluted and succussed to such a degree that no molecule of the original substance remains in the final medicine. It's a level of dilution that confounds conventional pharmacology – how can something so diluted still hold medicinal value? Scientists suggest the process imprints an energy signature or 'memory' from the original substance into the diluting medium, usually water or alcohol. This 'energized' preparation then resonates with the body, inducing a healing response.

Homeopathy perceives disease as a disturbance in our vital force, our inherent healing energy. It does not treat illnesses but patients, considering their physical symptoms, emotional states and life circumstances. Understanding a patient's unique symptom picture allows homeopaths to match a remedy to stimulate their vital force, enabling self-healing.

6.3. The Potent Power of Homeopathic Remedies

Homeopathic medicines, known as remedies, come in various potencies. Lower potencies (e.g., 6C or 30C) are generally used for acute, self-limiting conditions. Higher potencies (200C, 1M, 10M) are usually reserved for constitutional treatment – addressing deep-seated chronic conditions, often involving emotional or mental symptoms.

A well-selected homeopathic remedy resonates with the person's disease pattern and stimulates the body to correct the imbalance. This stimulation fosters a healing response, encouraging the body to heal itself.

6.4. Flower Essences: Gentle Solutions to Emotional Imbalances

Introduced by Dr. Edward Bach in the 20th century, who believed that physical illnesses had emotional causes, flower essences are dilutions of flower material developed to address profound issues of emotional health, soul development, and mind-body health.

Bach developed 38 flower remedies, each for a definable human emotional state, such as Fear, Uncertainty, Loneliness, Despondency or Despair, Over-sensitivity to influences and ideas, and Insufficient interest in present circumstances. Further remedies have been developed by different practitioners worldwide, exploring the healing potential of various flora.

Emotion is fundamentally energetic. Negative emotions can create energy blockages leading to physical illness. Flower essences, also energetic in nature, can help to clear such blockages, promoting physical healing indirectly.

6.5. How Do Flower Essences Work?

Flower essences work by the principle of resonance within the body's energy system, also known as life force, chi, or prana. They act as a catalyst for changes at a deep, subconscious level, helping us to change emotional attitudes that may be causing or exacerbating illness.

Each flower essence encompasses the positive, balancing energy of a specific emotion. Introducing this energy allows the body and mind to 'resonate' with it, gradually reducing or eliminating the negative emotion.

The subtlety and gentleness of flower essences make them particularly useful for sensitive individuals, children, and animals. They are also beneficial for anyone facing stress, grief, or mood-related challenges.

6.6. The Healing Duo: Homeopathy and Flower Essences

Homeopathy and flower essences may be used together in a complementary fashion. While homeopathy is generally directed at a person's overall symptom pattern, helping to stimulate the body's healing response, flower essences act at a subtle, emotional level.

Both modalities honour the unique individuality of each person and share a similar philosophy - invoking the body's self-healing mechanism. They respect the delicate interplay between mind, body, and spirit in the pathogenesis (disease formation) and healing processes.

Understanding and utilizing these gentle, nature-derived modalities can empower individuals on their path to wellness. Their capacity to catalyze healing responses at multiple, interconnected levels of our being offers a comprehensive, holistic approach to health and well-being.

While it is advised to consult with trained professionals for severe or chronic symptoms, everyone can benefit from learning and utilizing these gentle healers in daily life. They can be particularly beneficial for self-care, personal development, stress management, and preventive health care.

Homeopathy and flower essences invite us to deepen our relationship with the natural world, recognising the potent healing it offers. They serve as bridges, connecting us to our innate wisdom and the healing power of nature - nature's gentle healers indeed.

Chapter 7. Energy Healing: Breathing Life into Wellness

As we embark on our diverse voyage through the realm of alternative therapies, energy healing demands particular attention. Energy healing – the often ethereal, seemingly inaccessible domain where health and wellbeing root in the unseen currents of life — has been an integral part of healing traditions around the globe. It is a sphere where the science of the palpable realm converges with the esoteric wisdom of ages. So let's delve into the world of energy healing with a focus on one gem in its treasure chest — breathing, the unassuming yet potent channel of life energy.

7.1. Understanding Life Energy

Life energy — known by many names, such as "chi" in Chinese, "prana" in Sanskrit, or "ki" in Japanese — is believed to be the vital force that permeates all life. Ancient cultures built on this concept, developing healing practices aimed at balancing this energy to foster health and well-being. Modern science is increasingly resonating with this view, emphasizing the role of stress responses, emotions, and thought patterns — various facets of 'energy' — in our physiological functioning.

7.2. Energy Healing: The Breath Connection

Breathing is the most direct, conscious way we interact with our life energy. Notice how your breath changes when you're afraid, angry, or relaxed. Breath, as a bridge between the conscious and unconscious realms, offers us a unique portal to healing by modulating physiological responses and calming the mind.

7.3. The Principles of Breathwork

Breathwork employs varied breathing techniques to optimize physical health, emotional stability, and spiritual growth. The principles are rooted in three key aspects:

1. Conscious Awareness: Becoming mindful of your breathing shifts your focus from outside stimuli to your internal state. This, in turn, promotes relaxation and a deeper connection to your body.

2. Intentional Technique: Breathwork may involve unique patterns of inhalation, exhalation, and breath holding, often synchronized with body movements or visualizations.

3. Energetic Alignment: The process often aims at releasing energy blockages, improving energy flow and aligning the body's energy centers.

7.4. Deep Breathing

The simplest yet powerful breathwork technique, deep breathing requires you to breathe low into your belly, drawing more oxygen than shallow, chest-level breaths. This kind of diaphragmatic breathing initiates a relaxation response, slowing your heartbeat, lowering your blood pressure, and easing your stress response.

7.5. Box Breathing

Box Breathing, practiced by Navy Seals to manage stress in extreme situations, involves equal durations of inhale, hold, exhale, and hold. This pattern creates a sense of balance and has been reported to improve focus and performance.

7.6. 4-7-8 Breathing

The 4-7-8 breathing technique by Dr. Andrew Weil leans on ancient yogic traditions. It involves inhaling for four counts, holding the breath for seven, and exhaling with a whooshing sound for eight.

7.7. Pranayama

Pranayama, an integral part of yoga, leverages the breath to balance the body's energy systems. Techniques like Nadi Shodhana (alternate nostril breathing), Kapalabhati (forceful exhales and passive inhales), and Bhramari (bee breath), each serve specific healing purposes.

7.8. Synchronized Breathwork

Certain approaches, like Holotropic Breathwork developed by psychiatrist Stanislav Grof, involve vigorous rhythmic breathing that can facilitate emotional release. Often, this is practiced in a group setting accompanied by evocative music.

7.9. Breathwork for Health, Healing and Beyond

Breathwork offers numerous health benefits — from regulating autonomic nervous system responses, improving cardiovascular health, aiding digestion, to boosting immunity. On a psychological level, it can aid in releasing suppressed emotions, anxiety, and stress. Many have found it a path to profound spiritual experiences, connecting them with a deeper self or a sense of universal unity.

7.10. The Future of Breathing in Energy Healing

As we deepen our understanding of the profound links between our body, mind, emotions, and energy, Breathwork stands as a promising field. Ongoing research is exploring its potential in managing various health issues, mental health problems, and its synergistic role in boosting the effects of other therapies.

In this journey exploring the link between breathwork and energy healing, we find that breath, in its simplicity and depth, offers an exciting avenue to wellness. It shows us that each inhale offers an opportunity to draw vitality from the universe, each exhale a chance to release and renew. Embracing these principles indeed breathes life into wellness. As we welcome these practices into our lives, we open doors to holistic well-being, unearthing an inner harmony long forgotten in the rhythms of modern life.

Breathwork, in its myriad forms, is a key tool in our wellness toolbox. By understanding the capabilities of our breath, this seemingly automatic and overlooked process serves as a vital bridge spanning the conscious and unconscious, the physical and spiritual, the visible and the invisible aspects of our being. As we harness the power of breath, an element so basic yet so profound, we truly begin to grasp the magic that energy healing offers. Each breath becomes a step further into our journey of wellness — a journey towards aligning, harmonizing, and celebrating our existence in this dynamic dance of life.

Chapter 8. Transformative Power of Meditation and Mindfulness

Meditation and mindfulness have been practiced for thousands of years, across diverse cultures and societies. These practices encompass a vast array of techniques, but they all converge upon a singular intention: cultivation of attentive awareness and fostering inner peace.

8.1. Basics of Meditation and Mindfulness

To understand the transformative power of mindfulness and meditation, it's first crucial to understand their fundamental aspects. Mindfulness refers to the ability to be fully present, being aware of where we are and what we're doing, without becoming overly reactive or overwhelmed by what's happening around us. Meditation is a broader term that encompasses the application of certain techniques, such as focusing the mind on a particular object, thought, or activity, to train attention and awareness and achieve clarity and emotional calmness.

Does this entail merely sitting silently in a cross-legged position for long extended periods? No, mindfulness and meditation can be much more versatile, adaptable to your lifestyle and comfort. You can practice mindfulness at every moment, whether you're eating, driving, or engaging in your daily tasks.

8.2. The Neuroscience Behind Meditation and Mindfulness

The power of these activities lies in their ability to actually change the structure and function of our brains – a concept known as neuroplasticity. Recent neuroscientific research has shown the following impacts due to meditation and mindfulness practice:

- Increased gray matter density in areas responsible for learning, memory processing, and emotion regulation.

- Decreased gray matter density in the amygdala, responsible for stress and anxiety.

- Improved connectivity between brain regions.

- Enhanced focussed attention and cognitive flexibility.

This evidence from neuroscience adds a fresh dimension to our understanding of the transformative power of mindfulness and meditation, providing empirical support to what practitioners have experienced personally.

8.3. Techniques for Practice

Though mindfulness and meditation share common roots, there's a wide variety of techniques and methods within these practices. Few of them includes:

- Focused Attention Meditation: The practitioner focuses on a single item, such as your breath, a mantra, or a particular object.

- Body Scan or Progressive Relaxation: A method accessible to even mindfulness beginners. This involves slowly tightening and then relaxing one muscle group at a time throughout the body.

- Loving-Kindness Meditation: Also known as Metta meditation, its goal is to cultivate an attitude of love and kindness towards everything, even stressors or adversaries.

You may explore these methods and find those that resonate the most with your personality and lifestyle. Sometimes, it may involve trial and error, but the journey of discovery can be enriching in itself.

8.4. Mindfulness in Daily Life

While formal meditation has its advantages, an equally important aspect is bringing mindfulness to every moment of our daily life. Whether you are engaged in eating, washing dishes, or a tense conversation, bring your full attention to the task at hand. Practicing mindfulness daily can bring profound transformations in our relationship with our thoughts, emotions, and overall life experiences.

In conclusion, the transformative power of mindfulness and meditation lies not only in their potential to bring about changes in our minds and bodies, but also their ability to bring about a fundamental shift in our perspective towards life. While the journey can be intense and demanding, the rewards - tranquility, mental clarity, emotional equilibrium - are beyond measure. Embrace the transformative power of mindfulness and meditation, and embark on a journey towards a more peaceful, harmonious self.

Chapter 9. The Healing Magic of Herbs and Spices

For thousands of years, humans have turned to the bountiful gifts of nature for holistic remedies. Herbs and spices, each imbued with distinct characteristics and healing properties, have remained an integral component of this journey to wellness. This chapter takes an in-depth exploration into the healing magic inherent in these diverse plants.

9.1. The Historical Use of Herbs and Spices

Herbs and spices played profound roles in human history, serving as essential ingredients for culinary, medicinal, and even spiritual practices. Archaeologists have unearthed evidence of medicinal herb usage dating back to the Paleolithic age. Egyptian hieroglyphics illustrate herb cultivation, while ancient Chinese and Ayurvedic texts document extensive pharmacopeias delineating the uses of numerous herbs and spices.

Herbs such as mint, chamomile, and lavender were used in the Roman Empire to promote healing and longevity, with soldiers often carrying herb sacks for immediate use in the battlefield. During the Middle Ages, herb gardens were staple features in monastic orders, where monks would carefully cultivate and study these plants for their healing properties.

In the East, Ayurveda, the ancient Indian medicine system, utilized a broad array of herbs and spices such as turmeric, holy basil, and ashwagandha, believing these elements balance the doshas – the biological energies derived from the elements. On the other hand, traditional Chinese medicine interprets herbs and spices under the shí Zhen food theory, classifying them based on their yin (cooling) or yang (warming) properties.

9.2. Understanding the Healing Properties of Herbs and Spices

We look up to herbs and spices for their strong natural healing potential – veering from mere folklore and backed by modern scientific research. They contain plant compounds called phytochemicals, biologically active substances that can nourish, detoxify, and rebalance the body. Herbs such as echinacea, astragalus, and elderberry are known for their immune-boosting capabilities. In contrast, spices like turmeric and black pepper are recognized for their anti-inflammatory and antioxidant properties.

Let's delve into some ubiquitous herbs and spices.

9.2.1. Turmeric

Turmeric, a bright yellow spice essential in Indian cuisine, boasts a rich history of medicinal use spanning nearly 4,000 years. Revered in Ayurvedic medicine, turmeric is known for its compound curcumin, offering potent anti-inflammatory and antioxidant properties.

Studies suggest that curcumin can inhibit the production of inflammation-causing molecules, providing relief in various conditions like rheumatoid arthritis and inflammatory bowel disease. Moreover, turmeric has anticarcinogenic potentials backed by numerous scientific studies. It has shown promise in preventing the growth of cancer cells and enhancing the effect of chemotherapy.

To maximize the absorption of curcumin, it's advised to combine it with black pepper, which contains piperine, a compound known to enhance curcumin absorption by up to 2,000%.

9.2.2. Holy Basil

Considered a sacred plant in Hinduism, Holy Basil or "Tulsi" is an adaptogen. Adaptogens are a special class of herbs that aid in adapting to stress and promote or restore normal physiological functions.

Studies on Holy Basil show its effectiveness in relieving physical and mental stress, enhancing mood, and improving cognitive functions. It also holds antidiabetic properties, helping reduce blood sugar levels. The eugenol, rosmarinic acid, and other antioxidant compounds present help fortify the immune system, reduce inflammation, and combat premature aging.

9.2.3. Garlic

Garlic, a staple in many world cuisines, yields a plethora of health benefits. Its bioactive compound, allicin, possesses potent antibacterial, antiviral, and antifungal properties. Garlic is also an excellent cardiac ally, known to lower blood pressure, reduce LDL cholesterol levels, and prevent atherosclerosis.

Regular consumption of garlic may offer protection against certain types of cancer, thanks to its antioxidant content and anti-inflammatory properties. Additionally, garlic has been used for centuries to boost the immune system, fight colds, and treat a range of infections.

9.3. Including Herbs and Spices in Your Diet

While it's apparent how herbs and spices can positively impact our health, understanding how to include them in the diet remains key to unlocking their full healing potential.

Incorporating herbs and spices into your diet doesn't necessitate drastic changes in food habits. Simple techniques can markedly increase their presence in your daily meals:

- Turmeric can be added to smoothies, used to season roasted vegetables, or steeped with milk and honey for a comforting turmeric latte.

- Holy Basil leaves can be brewed into a calming tea or added to stir-fry vegetable dishes. They're also a flavorful addition to salads and soups.

- Garlic imparts richness to many dishes. It can be sautéed with vegetables, used to flavor meats, or consumed raw for a potent health boost.

Remember, while herbs and spices offer many health advantages, they are most effective when combined with an overall balanced diet and a healthy lifestyle.

9.4. Precautions and Side Effects

While notably beneficial, certain herbs and spices may not be suitable for everyone, especially when consumed in large amounts. For instance, turmeric can interfere with anticoagulants and cause stomach upset in some people. Holy Basil might affect fertility and is not recommended for pregnant women. Garlic can also thin the blood and interfere with certain medications.

It's vital to educate oneself on the potential side effects of herbs and spices and always consult healthcare professionals before incorporating these into your diet, especially if you are pregnant, nursing, or have a chronic health condition.

9.5. Conclusion

The natural world abounds with remedies waiting to be discovered, and herbs and spices stand as testament to this treasure. These plants represent a vibrant connection to our past, granting us the wisdom of the ages and a more holistic, natural approach to wellness. As we continue to understand the intricate links between diet and health, incorporating herbs and spices into our meals can not only complement the taste but also promises profound health benefits.

Chapter 10. Yoga, Tai Chi, and Reiki: Harmony in Movement

In seeking holistic wellness, we must turn our focus towards practices that integrate the body, mind, and spirit. Such harmonious integration provided by Yoga, Tai Chi, and Reiki, illuminates the path to health and wellbeing. Each practice, while unique, cultivates balance through the interplay of movement, meditation, and energy work.

10.1. Yoga: Union of Body, Mind, and Spirit

For thousands of years, Yoga has been a primary route for those seeking holistic healing and wellness. Originating in ancient India, this practice is much more than a physical exercise. It's a spiritual discipline designed to cultivate deep inner peace and self-awareness, uniting the physical body, the mind, and the spirit.

The practice of Yoga comprises several aspects: Asanas (poses), Pranayama (conscious control of breath), Dhyana (meditation), and Yamas and Niyamas (ethical and moral guidelines). Each of these elements contributes significantly towards improving our bodily strength, flexibility, mental clarity, emotional resilience, and spiritual growth.

```
Practicing Yoga regularly results in numerous health
benefits.

[cols=",,",]
|===
| Benefit | Explanation
| Physical health | Enhances muscular strength, promotes
```

flexibility, improves postural alignment, boosts
cardiovascular health, aids digestion, and improves
respiratory function.
| Mental health | Helps manage stress, reduces anxiety,
and fosters mindfulness.
| Emotional health | Inspires self-acceptance, nurtures
self-love, improves mood, and boosts self-esteem.
| Spiritual health | Encourages personal growth, fosters
connection with the universe, and cultivates inner
peace.
|===

Successful Yoga practice requires a calm and peaceful
environment, a comfortable Yoga mat, appropriate attire,
and a dedicated time for practice. It's crucial to
listen to your body and modify the poses as required.
And lastly, regular practice combined with genuine
dedication is the key to developing a profound Yoga
journey that cultivates holistic wellbeing.

=== Tai Chi: The Graceful Dance of Energy

Tai Chi is often depicted as a series of slow, fluid
movements performed gracefully. This ancient Chinese
martial art, renowned for its health benefits, is
practiced both for defense training and its therapeutic
implications. The principle embodying Tai Chi is the
pursuit of balance, expressed in the concept of Yin and
Yang -- these opposites illustrate the interplay of
opposing forces and harmonious existence.

The essence of Tai Chi lies within the graceful
movements, or "forms," which are meant to stimulate the
flow of qi (life force energy) throughout the body. By

performing these movements with mindful attention, the practitioner aims to achieve physical balance and harmony, thereby promoting overall health and wellness.

Just like Yoga, Tai Chi also offers diverse benefits:

[cols=",,",]
|===
| Benefit | Explanation
| Physical health | Enhances flexibility, improves muscle strength, aids in correcting poor postural or movement patterns, and benefits heart health.
| Mental health | Enhances concentration and cognitive abilities, reduces stress, and promotes relaxation.
| Emotional health | Encourages emotional stability, boosts mood, and provides a sense of peace and tranquility.
| Spiritual health | Facilitates a deeper understanding of oneself and the universe, centring on the interplay of physical and spiritual elements.
|===

As a beginner, it's recommended to begin with shorter routines, gradually increasing the duration as your endurance improves. Practicing Tai Chi requires loose, comfortable clothing and ample space for movement. Lastly, practicing Tai Chi with mindfulness, focusing on breath control and the flow of movements, is crucial in attaining its therapeutic benefits.

=== Reiki: The Life-Force Synchronizer

Reiki, originally from Japan, is an alternative therapy
that involves the transfer of universal energy from the
practitioner's palms to their patient. Increased life
force, or "Ki," is believed to enable self-healing, a
state of equilibrium, and a sense of wellbeing.

Receiving Reiki involves the practitioner placing their
hands lightly on or over specific areas of the
recipient's body to facilitate the flow of energy. These
techniques aim to treat the body, emotions, mind, and
spirit, producing many beneficial effects such as
relaxation and feelings of peace, security, and well-
being.

The potential benefits of Reiki are vast:

[cols=",,",]
|===
| Benefit | Explanation
| Physical health | Potentially accelerates body's self-
healing ability, aids better sleep, reduces blood
pressure, and helps relieve pain.
| Mental health | Assists in relieving stress, aids in
better focus and clarity, and augments learning, memory
and mental clarity.
| Emotional health | Cleans and clears emotions, helping
them to be more balanced and less dominated by fear and
doubt.
| Spiritual health | Connects with the higher self,
expanding consciousness and promoting spiritual growth.
|===

Reiki therapy can be learned and practiced by anyone. It offers an opportunity to take personal responsibility for maintaining health and treating ailments. An essential part of practicing Reiki is daily self-treatment, to strengthen the mind and body.

In closing, Yoga, Tai Chi, and Reiki each offer unique paths towards the common goal of wellness. While their practices differ significantly, they all spotlight the fundamental concept of the interconnectedness of body, mind, and spirit. Engaging in these practices allows us the opportunity to cultivate inner peace, promote physical health, and enhance spiritual growth.

== The Future of Holistic Health: Integrative Medicine and Beyond
Holistic health, or the approach that emphasizes the entire person, including physical, mental, emotional, and spiritual aspects of their life, continues to gain traction in contemporary society. This unwavering momentum is signaling a vital shift in how we understand and attend to our health. The keen observation of human nature tells us that our health is not just the absence of disease but an amalgamation of countless factors intricately woven into our life's tapestry. As we gaze into the future of holistic health, we're presented with an exciting panorama of emerging trends, therapies, and philosophical shifts; a future where the holistic health paradigm forms the bedrock of our healthcare system and a vision that recognizes the interconnectedness of body, mind, spirit, and environment.

=== Evolving Holistic Perspective

The holistic perspective on health and healing has been

part of our collective wisdom since ancient times, with principles echoing in traditional Chinese medicine and Ayurveda, the Indian system of medicine. It is an understanding that thrives on the notion that the mind, body, and spirit are intimately connected and that the health of one affects the health of the others. Irrespective of cultural context, traditional healing systems have always revered this holistic view, tending not only to the physical symptoms of illness but also providing intense care to psychological, social, and spiritual realms. The future of holistic health appears to be headed in a much similar direction, revitalizing these time-honored viewpoints and integrating them seamlessly within our modern healthcare milieu.

=== Integrative Medicine: The Future is Now

This quote from the academic and scholar Rachel Naomi Remen best encapsulates the essence of integrative medicine, "At its core, healing is a process that happens on an invisible level. It happens within a human being and it is a process by which people reclaim the level of integrity and wholeness necessary for their well-being." Integrative medicine's future emphasizes optimizing health and wellness across a person's lifespan, rather than merely managing diseases.

Integrative medicine represents an exciting departure from assembly-line medicine, incorporating a broad range of both conventional and complementary therapies. The core philosophy subtly blends modern science with the wisdom of ancient healing traditions. Unlike the stringent dichotomy between conventional and alternative treatments, integrative medicine champions a more inclusive, patient-centered approach—the convergence point of the best of all therapeutic worlds. It

emphasizes a therapeutic relationship, promoting health
and wellness encompassing a person's physical, mental,
spiritual, and environmental influences.

=== Holistic Innovations: Personalized Medicine

At the forefront of medicine's future is personalized
medicine—a cutting-edge, scientific approach with the
promise of revolutionizing healthcare. By leveraging
genetic analysis and other diagnostic tools,
personalized therapies assure targeted, individualized
treatment plans tailored to a person's unique genetic
makeup, lifestyle, and environment. In doing so, it
creates a synchrony where the principle of
individualized care, a tenet central to holistic
healing, is integrated with high-tech scientific
discovery.

Although considered a relatively new concept,
personalized medicine is setting the groundwork for many
potential benefits. It holds enormous potential in the
subtle shift of medicine—from primarily reactive to a
proactive, predictive, and preventive approach. This
shift resonates strongly with the underlying principles
of holistic health and presents itself as the key to
unlocking a future where holistic health becomes
mainstream healthcare.

=== The Emergence of Mind-Body Therapies

One of the significant narratives in the future of
holistic health is the growing respect for mind-body
therapies. Practices like mindfulness, meditation, yoga,
and biofeedback tell a compelling story about the
inseparability of physical and mental health,
reaffirming the notion that our thoughts, beliefs, and

emotions substantially impact our health. With
progressive strides in neuroscience and technology, the
connection between the mind and body is becoming more
evident, indicating a bright future of holistic health
illuminated with improved mental well-being.

=== The Potential of Functional Medicine

The holistic health landscape is being further
diversified with the emergence of functional medicine.
It's a system-oriented approach, engaging both patient
and practitioner in a therapeutic partnership.
Functional medicine emphasizes understanding the root
cause of disease—addressing the 'why' rather than 'what'
of the ailment. The future of holistic health lies in
embracing such comprehensive strategies in contemporary
care, where we no longer just manage symptoms but rather
target the root problems and address them using multi-
modal therapeutic approaches.

=== The Rise of Natural and Plant-based Medicine

The future of holistic health also gleams with nature's
brilliance. Medicinal plants, traditional natural
therapies, and natural bioactive compounds are gaining
recognition in managing ailments—ranging from common
illnesses to chronic conditions. Natural and plant-based
therapies carve out a future where holistic approaches
meet rigorous scientific validation, fostering healthier
communities and ecosystems.

=== Embracing the Digital Realm: eHealth and
Telemedicine

Possibilities abound when we wed holistic health
concepts and digital technology—telemedicine and eHealth

are just the start. Digital health interventions offer
real-time health monitoring, AI-assisted diagnostics,
virtual wellness coaching, and much more. Telemedicine
and eHealth stand as marquees of medical
democratization, allowing individuals in remote areas to
receive healthcare, reducing the need for hospital
visits, and providing healthcare at the convenience of
home. While this integration drives the narrative for
better accessibility and inclusivity, it also extends
the reach of holistic health and wellness in
unprecedented ways.

The era of holistic health is well underway, promising
an exciting epoch of integrative medicine and beyond.
Technological advancements, therapeutic innovation, and
shifts in our understanding of health are intersecting
at a unique juncture. The underlying resurgence of age-
old wisdom, intertwined with high-tech science, opens
new pathways to health and well-being, presenting a
vision of holistic health that is as profound as it is
powerful. As we continue to explore this evolving
landscape, it becomes clear that holistic health's
future holds the promise of a healthcare revolution—one
that honors the individual at the core of care, values
the symbiosis of mind and body, and appreciates our
fundamental kinship with nature.